Global Initiative for Chronic Obstructive Lung Disease

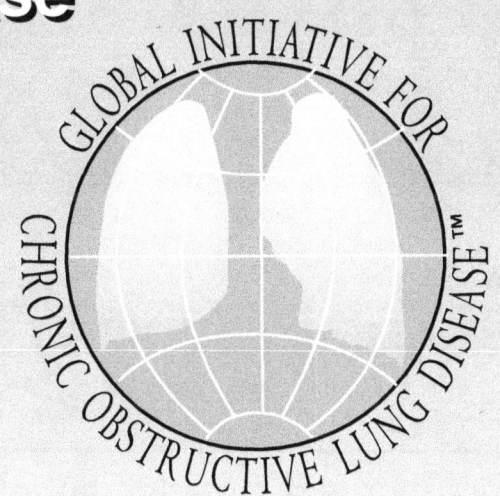

POCKET GUIDE TO
COPD DIAGNOSIS, MANAGEMENT, AND PREVENTION

A Guide for Health Care Professionals

UPDATED 2016

Global Initiative for Chronic Obstructive Lung Disease

Pocket Guide to COPD Diagnosis, Management and Prevention, Updated 2016

GOLD Board of Directors

Marc Decramer, MD, Chair
University of Leuven
Leuven, Belgium

Alvar G. Agusti, MD
Universitat de Barcelona
Barcelona, Spain

Jean Bourbeau, MD
McGill University Health Centre
Montreal, Quebec, Canada

Bartolome R. Celli, MD
Brigham and Women's Hospital
Boston, Massachusetts, US

Rongchang Chen, MD
Guangzhou Institute of Respiratory Disease
Guangzhou, PRC

Gerard Criner, MD
Temple University School of Medicine
Philadelphia, Pennsylvania, US

Peter Frith, MD
Repatriation General Hospital, Adelaide
South Australia, Australia

David Halpin, MD
Royal Devon and Exeter Hospital
Devon, UK

M.Victorina López Varela, MD
Universidad de la República
Montevideo, Uruguay

Masaharu Nishimura, MD
Hokkaido Univ School of Medicine
Sapporo, Japan

Claus Vogelmeier, MD
University of Gießen and Marburg
Marburg, Germany

GOLD Science Committee

Jørgen Vestbo, MD, *Denmark, UK, Chair*
Alvar Agusti, MD, *Spain*
Antonio Anzueto, MD, *USA*
Marc Decramer, MD, *Belgium*
Leonardo M. Fabbri, MD, *Italy*
Fernando Martinez, MD, *USA*

Nicolas Roche, MD, *France*
Roberto Rodriguez Roisin, MD, *Spain*
Donald Sin, MD, *Canada*
Dave Singh, MD, *UK*
Robert A. Stockley, MD, *UK*
Jadwiga A. Wedzicha, MD, *UK*

GOLD Science Director
Suzanne Hurd, PhD, *USA*

GOLD National Leaders

Representatives from many countries serve as a network for the dissemination and implementation of programs for diagnosis, management, and prevention of COPD. The GOLD Board of Directors is grateful to the many GOLD National Leaders who participated in discussions of concepts that appear in GOLD reports.

TABLE OF CONTENTS

INTRODUCTION

Chronic Obstructive Pulmonary Disease (COPD) is a major cause of morbidity and mortality throughout the world. Much has been learned about COPD since the Global Initiative for Chronic Obstructive Lung Disease issued its first report, *Global Strategy for the Diagnosis, Management, and Prevention of COPD*, in 2001. Treatment of COPD is now aimed at immediately relieving and reducing the impact of symptoms, as well as reducing the risk of future adverse health events such as exacerbations. These dual goals emphasize the need for clinicians to maintain a focus on both the short-term and long-term impact of COPD on their patients. A framework for COPD management that matches individualized assessment of the disease to these treatment objectives will better meet each patient's needs.

Several educational tools and publications oriented around this approach to COPD are available at http://www.goldcopd.org and can be adapted to local health care systems and resources:

- *Global Strategy for the Diagnosis, Management, and Prevention of COPD*. Scientific information and recommendations for COPD programs. (Updated 2016)
- *Executive Summary, Global Strategy for the Diagnosis, Management, and Prevention of COPD. Am J Respir Crit* Care Med. 2013 Feb 15;187(4):347-65.
- *Pocket Guide to COPD Diagnosis, Management, and Prevention.* Summary of patient care information for primary health care professionals. (Updated 2016)
- *What You and Your Family Can Do About COPD.* Information booklet for patients and their families.

This Pocket Guide has been developed from the *Global Strategy for the Diagnosis, Management, and Prevention of COPD* (Updated 2016). Technical discussions of COPD and COPD management, evidence levels, and specific citations from the scientific literature are included in that source document.

KEY POINTS

- **Chronic Obstructive Pulmonary Disease (COPD)**, a common preventable and treatable disease, is characterized by persistent airflow limitation that is usually progressive and associated with an enhanced chronic inflammatory response in the airways and the lung to noxious particles or gases. Exacerbations and comorbidities contribute to the overall severity in individual patients.

- Worldwide, the most commonly encountered risk factor for COPD is **tobacco smoking.** Other types of tobacco, (e.g. pipe, cigar, water pipe) and marijuana are also risk factors for COPD. In many countries, **outdoor, occupational, and indoor air pollution** – the latter resulting from the burning of biomass fuels – are also major COPD risk factors.

- A **clinical diagnosis** of COPD should be considered in any patient who has dyspnea, chronic cough or sputum production, and a history of exposure to risk factors for the disease. Spirometry is required to make the diagnosis in this clinical context.

- **Assessment** of COPD is based on the patient's symptoms, risk of exacerbations, the severity of the spirometric abnormality, and the identification of comorbidities.

- Appropriate **pharmacologic therapy** can reduce COPD symptoms, reduce the frequency and severity of exacerbations, and improve health status and exercise tolerance.

- All COPD patients with breathlessness when walking at their own pace on level ground appear to benefit from **rehabilitation** and maintenance of **physical activity**.

- An **exacerbation** of COPD is an acute event characterized by a worsening of the patient's respiratory symptoms that is beyond normal day-to-day variations and leads to a change in medication.

- COPD often **coexists with other diseases (comorbidities)** that may have a significant impact on prognosis.

WHAT IS CHRONIC OBSTRUCTIVE PULMONARY DISEASE (COPD)?

Chronic Obstructive Pulmonary Disease (COPD), a common preventable and treatable disease, is characterized by persistent airflow limitation that is usually progressive and associated with an enhanced chronic inflammatory response in the airways and the lung to noxious particles or gases. Exacerbations and comorbidities contribute to the overall severity in individual patients.

This definition does not use the terms chronic bronchitis and emphysema* and excludes asthma (reversible airflow limitation).

Symptoms of COPD include:

- Dyspnea

- Chronic cough

- Chronic sputum production

Episodes of acute worsening of these symptoms (exacerbations) often occur.

Spirometry is required to make a clinical diagnosis of COPD; the presence of a post-bronchodilator $FEV_1/FVC < 0.70$ confirms the presence of persistent airflow limitation and thus of COPD.

---

*Chronic bronchitis, defined as the presence of cough and sputum production for at least 3 months in each of 2 consecutive years, is not necessarily associated with airflow limitation. Emphysema, defined as destruction of the alveoli, is a pathological term that is sometimes (incorrectly) used clinically and describes only one of several structural abnormalities present in patients with COPD – but can also be found in subjects with normal lung function.

WHAT CAUSES COPD?

Worldwide, the most commonly encountered risk factor for COPD is **tobacco smoking**. Other types of tobacco, (e.g. pipe, cigar, water pipe) and marijuana are also risk factors for COPD. Outdoor, occupational, and indoor air pollution – the latter resulting from the burning of biomass fuels – are other major COPD risk factors. Nonsmokers may also develop COPD.

The genetic risk factor that is best documented is a severe hereditary deficiency of alpha-1 antitrypsin. It provides a model for how other genetic risk factors are thought to contribute to COPD.

COPD risk is related to the total burden of inhaled particles a person encounters over their lifetime:

- **Tobacco smoke**, including cigarette, pipe, cigar, and other types of tobacco smoking popular in many countries, as well as environmental tobacco smoke (ETS)

- **Indoor air pollution** from biomass fuel used for cooking and heating in poorly vented dwellings, a risk factor that particularly affects women in developing countries

- **Occupational dusts and chemicals** (vapors, irritants, and fumes) when the exposures are sufficiently intense or prolonged

- **Outdoor air pollution** also contributes to the lungs' total burden of inhaled particles, although it appears to have a relatively small effect in causing COPD

In addition, any factor that affects lung growth during gestation and childhood (low birth weight, respiratory infections, etc.) has the potential to increase an individual's risk of developing COPD.

DIAGNOSIS OF COPD

A clinical diagnosis of COPD should be considered in any patient who has dyspnea, chronic cough or sputum production, and a history of exposure to risk factors for the disease (**Table 1**).

Table 1. Key Indicators for Considering a Diagnosis of COPD

Consider COPD, and perform spirometry, if any of these indicators are present in an individual over age 40. These indicators are not diagnostic themselves, but the presence of multiple key indicators increases the probability of a diagnosis of COPD. Spirometry is required to establish a diagnosis of COPD.

Dyspnea that is: Progressive (worsens over time).
Characteristically worse with exercise.
Persistent.

Chronic cough: May be intermittent and may be unproductive.

Chronic sputum production:
Any pattern of chronic sputum production may indicate COPD.

History of exposure to risk factors:
Tobacco smoke (including popular local preparations).
Smoke from home cooking and heating fuels.
Occupational dusts and chemicals.

Family history of COPD

Spirometry is required to make a clinical diagnosis of COPD; the presence of a postbronchodilator $FEV_1/FVC < 0.70$ confirms the presence of persistent airflow limitation and thus of COPD. All health care workers who care for COPD patients should have access to spirometry. **Appendix I: Spirometry for Diagnosis of Airflow Limitation in COPD** summarizes the lung function measurements that are key to making a spirometry diagnosis and details some of the factors needed to achieve accurate test results.

Differential Diagnosis: A major differential diagnosis is asthma. In some patients with chronic asthma, a clear distinction from COPD is not possible using current imaging and physiological testing techniques. In these patients, current management is similar to that of asthma. Other potential diagnoses are usually easier to distinguish from COPD (**Table 2**).

Table 2. COPD and its Differential Diagnoses

Diagnosis	Suggestive Features
COPD	Onset in mid-life. Symptoms slowly progressive. History of tobacco smoking or exposure to other types of smoke.
Asthma	Onset early in life (often childhood). Symptoms vary widely from day to day. Symptoms worse at night/early morning. Allergy, rhinitis, and/or eczema also present. Family history of asthma.
Congestive Heart Failure	Chest X-ray shows dilated heart, pulmonary edema. Pulmonary function tests indicate volume restriction, not airflow limitation.
Bronchiectasis	Large volumes of purulent sputum. Commonly associated with bacterial infection. Chest X-ray/CT shows bronchial dilation, bronchial wall thickening.
Tuberculosis	Onset all ages. Chest X-ray shows lung infiltrate. Microbiological confirmation. High local prevalence of tuberculosis.
Obliterative Bronchiolitis	Onset at younger age, nonsmokers. May have history of rheumatoid arthritis or acute fume exposure. Seen after lung or bone marrow transplantation. CT on expiration shows hypodense areas.
Diffuse Panbronchiolitis	Predominantly seen in patients of Asian descent. Most patients are male and nonsmokers. Almost all have chronic sinusitis. Chest X-ray and HRCT show diffuse small centrilobular nodular opacities and hyperinflation.

These features tend to be characteristic of the respective diseases, but are not mandatory. For example, a person who has never smoked may develop COPD (especially in the developing world where other risk factors may be more important than cigarette smoking); asthma may develop in adult and even in elderly patients.

ASSESSMENT OF COPD

The goals of COPD assessment are to determine the severity of the disease, its impact on patient's health status, and the risk of future events (exacerbations, hospital admissions, death) in order to guide therapy. Assess the following aspects of the disease separately:

- Symptoms
- Degree of airflow limitation (using spirometry)
- Risk of exacerbations
- Comorbidities

Assess Symptoms: Validated questionnaires such as the COPD Assessment Test (CAT) or the Clinical COPD Questionnaire (CCQ) are recommended for a comprehensive assessment of symptoms. The modified British Medical Research Council (mMRC) scale provides only an assessment of breathlessness.

Assess Degree of Airflow Limitation Using Spirometry: Table 3 provides the classification of airflow limitation severity in COPD.

Table 3. Classification of Severity of Airflow Limitation in COPD (Based on Post-Bronchodilator FEV_1)		
In patients with $FEV_1/FVC < 0.70$:		
GOLD 1:	Mild	$FEV_1 \geq 80\%$ predicted
GOLD 2:	Moderate	$50\% \leq FEV_1 < 80\%$ predicted
GOLD 3:	Severe	$30\% \leq FEV_1 < 50\%$ predicted
GOLD 4:	Very Severe	$FEV_1 < 30\%$ predicted

Assess Risk of Exacerbations: An exacerbation of COPD is defined as an acute event characterized by a worsening of the patient's respiratory symptoms that is beyond normal day-to-day variations and leads to a change in medication. The best predictor of having frequent exacerbations (2 or more per year) is a history of previous treated events. The risk of exacerbations also increases as airflow limitation worsens. Hospitalization for a COPD exacerbation is associated with a poor prognosis with increased risk of death.

Assess Comorbidities: Cardiovascular diseases, osteoporosis, depression and anxiety, skeletal muscle dysfunction, metabolic syndrome, and lung cancer among other diseases occur frequently in COPD patients. These comorbid conditions may influence mortality and hospitalizations, and should be looked for routinely and treated appropriately.

Combined Assessement of COPD: Table 4 provides a rubric for combining these assessments to improve management of COPD.

- **Symptoms:**
  Less Symptoms   (mMRC 0-1 or CAT < 10):   patient is (A) or (C)
  More Symptoms   (mMRC ≥ 2 or CAT ≥ 10):   patient is (B) or (D)

- **Airflow Limitation:**
  Low Risk   (GOLD 1 or 2):   patient is (A) or (B)
  High Risk   (GOLD 3 or 4):   patient is (C) or (D)

- **Exacerbations:**
  Low Risk: ≤ 1 per year *and* no hospitalization for exacerbation: patient is (A) or (B)
  High Risk: ≥ 2 per year *or* ≥ 1 with hospitalization: patient is (C) or (D)

Table 4. Combined Assessment of COPD
*When assessing risk, choose the **highest risk** according to GOLD grade or exacerbation history.*
(One or more hospitalizations for COPD exacerbations should be considered high risk.)

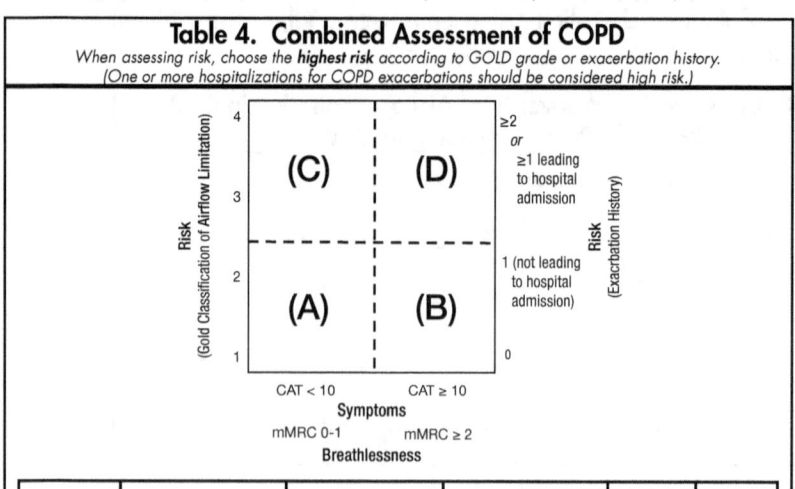

Patient	Characteristic	Spirometric Classification	Exacerbations per year	CAT	mMRC
A	Low Risk Less Symptoms	GOLD 1-2	≤ 1	< 10	0-1
B	Low Risk More Symptoms	GOLD 1-2	≤ 1	≥ 10	≥ 2
C	High Risk Less Symptoms	GOLD 3-4	≥ 2	< 10	0-1
D	High Risk More Symptoms	GOLD 3-4	≥ 2	≥ 10	≥ 2

THERAPEUTIC OPTIONS

Smoking cessation has the greatest capacity to influence the natural history of COPD. Health care providers should encourage all patients who smoke to quit.

- **Counseling** delivered by physicians and other health professionals significantly increases quit rates over self-initiated strategies. Even a brief (3-minute) period of counseling to urge a smoker to quit results in smoking quit rates of 5-10%.

- **Nicotine replacement therapy** (nicotine gum, inhaler, nasal spray, transdermal patch, sublingual tablet, or lozenge) as well as **pharmacotherapy** with varenicline, bupropion, or nortriptyline reliably increases long-term smoking abstinence rates and these treatments are significantly more effective than placebo.

Smoking Prevention: Encourage comprehensive tobacco-control policies and programs with clear, consistent, and repeated nonsmoking messages. Work with government officials to pass legislation to establish smoke-free schools, public facilities, and work environments and encourage patients to keep smoke-free homes.

Occupational Exposure: Emphasize primary prevention, which is best achieved by elimination or reduction of exposures to various substances in the workplace. Secondary prevention, achieved through surveillance and early detection, is also important.

Indoor and Outdoor Air Pollution: Implement measures to reduce or avoid indoor air pollution from burning biomass fuel for cooking and heating in poorly ventilated dwellings. Advise patients to monitor public announcements of air quality and, depending on the severity of their disease, avoid vigorous exercise outdoors or stay indoors during pollution episodes.

Physical Activity: All COPD patients benefit from regular physical activity and should repeatedly be encouraged to remain active.

PHARMACOLOGIC THERAPIES FOR STABLE COPD

Pharmacologic therapy is used to reduce symptoms, reduce the frequency and severity of exacerbations, and improve health status and exercise tolerance. Each treatment regimen needs to be patient-specific as the relationship between the severity of symptoms and the severity of airflow limitation is influenced by other factors, such as the frequency and severity of exacerbations, the presence of respiratory failure, comorbidities (cardiovascular disease, osteoporosis, etc.), and general health status. The classes of medications commonly used in treating COPD are shown in **Table 5**. The choice within each class depends on the availability of medication and the patient's response.

Bronchodilators: These medications are central to symptom management in COPD.

- Inhaled therapy is preferred.
- The choice between beta$_2$-agonists, anticholinergics, theophylline, or combination therapy depends on the availability of medications and each patient's individual response in terms of symptom relief and side effects.
- Bronchodilators are prescribed on an as-needed or on a regular basis to prevent or reduce symptoms.
- Long-acting inhaled bronchodilators are convenient and more effective at producing maintained symptom relief than short-acting bronchodilators.
- Long-acting inhaled bronchodilators reduce exacerbations and related hospitalizations and improve symptoms and health status, and tiotropium improves the effectiveness of pulmonary rehabilitation.
- Combining bronchodilators of different pharmacological classes may improve efficacy and decrease the risk of side effects compared to increasing the dose of a single bronchodilator.

Inhaled Corticosteroids: In COPD patients with FEV$_1$ < 60% predicted, regular treatment with inhaled corticosteroids improves symptoms, lung function, and quality of life, and reduces the frequency of exacerbations. Inhaled corticosteroid therapy is associated with an increased risk of pneumonia. Withdrawal from treatment with inhaled corticosteroids may lead to exacerbations in some patients. Long-term monotherapy with inhaled corticosteroids is not recommended.

Combination Inhaled Corticosteroid/Bronchodilator Therapy: An inhaled corticosteroid combined with a long-acting beta$_2$-agonist is more effective than either individual component in improving lung function and health status and reducing exacerbations in patients with moderate to very severe COPD. Combination therapy is associated with an increased risk of pneumonia. Addition of a long-acting beta$_2$-agonist/inhaled glucocorticosteroid to tiotropium appears to provide additional benefits.

Oral Corticosteroids: Long-term treatment with oral corticosteroids is not recommended.

Phosphodiesterase-4 inhibitors: In GOLD 3 and GOLD 4 patients with a history of exacerbations and chronic bronchitis, the phosphodiesterase-4 inhibitor roflumilast reduces exacerbations treated with oral corticosteroids. These effects are also seen when roflumilast is added to long-acting bronchodilators; there are no comparison studies with inhaled corticosteroids.

Methylxanthines. Methylxanthines are less effective and less well tolerated than inhaled long-acting bronchodilators and are not recommended if those drugs are available and affordable.   There is evidence for a modest bronchodilator effect and some symptomatic benefit of these medications compared with placebo in stable COPD.   Addition of theophylline to salmeterol produces a greater increase in FEV$_1$ and relief of breathlessness than salmeterol alone. Low-dose theophylline reduces exacerbations but does not improve post-bronchodilator lung function.

Other Pharmacologic Treatments

Vaccines: Influenza vaccines can reduce serious illness and death in COPD patients. Vaccines containing killed or live, inactivated viruses are recommended, and should be given once each year. Pneumococcal polysaccharide vaccine is recommended for COPD patients 65 years and older, and has been shown to reduce community-acquired pneumonia in those under age 65 with FEV$_1$ < 40% predicted.

Alpha-1 Antitrypsin Augmentation Therapy: Not recommended for patients with COPD that is unrelated to alpha-1 antitrypsin deficiency.

Antibiotics: Not recommended except for treatment of infectious exacerbations and other bacterial infections.

Table 5. Formulations and Typical Doses of COPD Medications*

Drug	Inhaler (mcg)	Solution for Nebulizer (mg/ml)	Oral	Vials for Injection (mg)	Duration of Action (hours)
Beta₂-agonists					
Short-acting					
Fenoterol	100-200 (MDI)	1	0.05% (Syrup)		4-6
Levalbuterol	45-90 (MDI)	0.21, 0.42			6-8
Salbutamol (albuterol)	100, 200 (MDI & DPI)	5	5 mg (Pill), 0.024%(Syrup)	0.1, 0.5	4-6
Terbutaline	400, 500 (DPI)		2.5, 5 mg (Pill)		4-6
Long-acting					
Formoterol	4.5-12 (MDI & DPI)	0.01¶			12
Arformoterol		0.0075			12
Indacaterol	75-300 (DPI)				24
Olodaterol	5mcg (SMI)				24
Salmeterol	25-50 (MDI & DPI)				12
Tulobuterol			2 mg (transdermal)		24
Anticholinergics					
Short-acting					
Ipratropium bromide	20, 40 (MDI)	0.25-0.5			6-8
Oxitropium bromide	100 (MDI)	1.5			7-9
Long-acting					
Aclidinium bromide	322 (DPI)				12
Glycopyrronium bromide	44 (DPI)				24
Tiotropium	18 (DPI), 5 (SMI)				24
Umeclidinium	62.5 (DPI)				24
Combination short-acting beta₂-agonist plus anticholinergic in one inhaler					
Fenoterol/Ipratropium	200/80 (MDI)	1.25/0.5			6-8
Salbutamol/Ipratropium	100/20 (SMI)				6-8
Combination long-acting beta₂-agonist plus anticholinergic in one inhaler					
Formoterol/aclidinium	12/340 (DPI)				12
Indacaterol/glycopyrronium	85/43 (DPI)				24
Olodaterol/tiotropium	5/5 (SMI)				24
Vilanterol/umeclidinium	25/62.5 (DPI)				24
Methylxanthines					
Aminophylline			200-600 mg (Pill)	240	Variable, up to 24
Theophylline (SR)			100-600 mg (Pill)		Variable, up to 24
Inhaled corticosteroids					
Beclomethasone	50-400 (MDI & DPI)	0.2-0.4			
Budesonide	100, 200, 400 (DPI)	0.20. 0.25, 0.5			
Fluticasone	50-500 (MDI & DPI)				
Combination long-acting beta₂-agonists plus corticosteroids in one inhaler					
Formoterol/beclometasone	6/100 (MDI & DPI)				
Formoterol/budesonide	4.5/160 (MDI) 9/320 (DPI)				
Formoterol/mometasone	10/200, 10/400 (MDI)				
Salmeterol/Fluticasone	50/100, 250, 500 (DPI)				
Vilanterol/Fluticasone furoate	25/100 (DPI)				
Systemic corticosteroids					
Prednisone			5-60 mg (Pill)		
Methyl-prednisolone			4, 8, 16 mg (Pill)		
Phosphodiesterase-4 inhibitors					
Roflumilast			500 mcg (Pill)		24

MDI=metered dose inhaler; DPI=dry powder inhaler; SMI=soft mist inhaler
*Not all formulations are available in all countries; in some countries, other formulations may be available.
¶Formoterol nebulized solution is based on the unit dose vial containing 20 mcg in a volume of 2.0 ml

14

Mucolytic Agents: Patients with viscous sputum may benefit from mucolytics (e.g. carbocysteine), but overall benefits are very small.

Antitussives: Use is not recommended.

Vasodilators: Nitric oxide is contraindicated in stable COPD. The use of endothelium-modulating agents for the treatment of pulmonary hypertension associated with COPD is not recommended.

OTHER TREATMENTS

Rehabilitation: Patients at all stages of disease benefit from exercise training programs with improvements in exercise tolerance and symptoms of dyspnea and fatigue. Benefits can be sustained even after a single pulmonary rehabilitation program. The minimum length of an effective rehabilitation program is 6 weeks; the longer the program continues, the more effective the results. Benefit does wane after a rehabilitation program ends, but if exercise training is maintained at home the patient's health status remains above pre-rehabilitation levels.

Oxygen Therapy: The long-term administration of oxygen (> 15 hours per day) to patients with chronic respiratory failure has been shown to increase survival in patients with severe, resting hypoxemia. Long-term oxygen therapy is indicated for patients who have:

- PaO_2 at or below 7.3 kPa (55 mmHg) or SaO_2 at or below 88%, with or without hypercapnia confirmed twice over a three-week period; *or*

- PaO_2 between 7.3 kPa (55 mmHg) and 8.0 kPa (60 mmHg), or SaO_2 of 88%, if there is evidence of pulmonary hypertension, peripheral edema suggesting congestive cardiac failure, or polycythemia (hematocrit > 55%).

Ventilatory Support: The combination of non-invasive ventilation with long-term oxygen therapy may be of some use in a selected subset of patients, particularly in those with pronounced daytime hypercapnia. It may improve survival but does not improve quality of life. There are clear benefits of continuous positive airway pressure (CPAP) on both survival and risk of hospital admission.

Surgical Treatments: The advantage of lung volume reduction surgery (LVRS) over medical therapy is more significant among patients with upper-lobe predominant emphysema and low exercise capacity prior to treatment, although LVRS is costly relative to health-care programs not including surgery. In appropriately selected patients with very severe COPD, lung transplantation has been shown to improve quality of life and functional capacity.

Non-surgical bronchoscopic lung volume reduction techniques should not be used outside clinical trials until more data are available.

Palliative Care, End-of-life Care, and Hospice Care: The disease trajectory in COPD is usually marked by a gradual decline in health status and increasing symptoms, punctuated by acute exacerbations that are associated with an increased risk of dying. Progressive respiratory failure, cardiovascular diseases, malignancies and other diseases are the primary cause of death in patients with COPD hospitalized for an exacerbation. Thus palliative care, end-of-life care, and hospice care are important components of the management of patients with advanced COPD.

MANAGEMENT OF STABLE COPD

Once COPD has been diagnosed, effective management should be based on an individualized assessment of current symptoms and future risks:

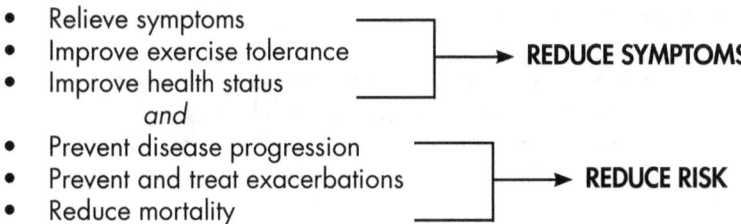

- Relieve symptoms
- Improve exercise tolerance ──→ **REDUCE SYMPTOMS**
- Improve health status
  and
- Prevent disease progression
- Prevent and treat exacerbations ──→ **REDUCE RISK**
- Reduce mortality

These goals should be reached with minimal side effects from treatment, a particular challenge in COPD patients because they commonly have comorbidities that also need to be carefully identified and treated.

NON-PHARMACOLOGIC TREATMENT

Non-pharmacologic management of COPD according to the individualized assessment of symptoms and exacerbation risk is shown in **Table 6**.

Table 6. Non-Pharmacologic Management of COPD

Patient Group	Essential	Recommended	Depending on Local Guidelines
A	Smoking cessation (can include pharmacologic treatment)	Physical activity	Flu vaccination Pneumococcal vaccination
B, C, D	Smoking cessation (can include pharmacologic treatment) Pulmonary rehabilitation	Physical activity	Flu vaccination Pneumococcal vaccination

PHARMACOLOGIC TREATMENT

A proposed model for initial pharmacological management of COPD according to the assessment of symptoms and risk (**Table 4**) is shown in **Table 7**.

Bronchodilators – Recommendations:

- For both beta$_2$-agonists and anticholinergics, long-acting formulations are preferred over short-acting formulations.
- The combined use of short- or long-acting beta$_2$-agonists and anticholinergics may be considered if symptoms are not improved with single agents.
- Based on efficacy and side effects, inhaled bronchodilators are preferred over oral bronchodilators.
- Based on evidence of relatively low efficacy and greater side effects, treatment with theophylline is not recommended unless other bronchodilators are not available or unaffordable for long-term treatment.

Corticosteroids and Phosphodiesterase-4 Inhibitors – Recommendations

- There is no evidence to recommend a short-term therapeutic trial with oral corticosteroids in patients with COPD to identify those who will respond to inhaled corticosteroids or other medications.
- Long-term treatment with inhaled corticosteroids is recommended for patients with severe and very severe airflow limitation and for patients with frequent exacerbations that are not adequately controlled by long-acting bronchodilators.
- Long-term monotherapy with oral corticosteroids is not recommended in COPD.
- Long-term monotherapy with inhaled corticosteroids is not recommended in COPD because it is less effective than the combination of inhaled corticosteroids with long-acting beta$_2$-agonists.
- Long-term treatment containing inhaled corticosteroids should not be prescribed outside their indications, due to the risk of pneumonia and the possibility of a slightly increased risk of fractures following long-term exposure.
- The phosphodiesterase-4 inhibitor roflumilast may also be used to reduce exacerbations for patients with chronic bronchitis, severe and very severe airflow limitation, and frequent exacerbations that are not adequately controlled by long-acting bronchodilators.

Table 7: Pharmacologic Therapy for Stable COPD*

Patient Group	RECOMMENDED FIRST CHOICE	ALTERNATIVE CHOICE	OTHER POSSIBLE TREATMENTS**
A	SA anticholinergic prn or SA beta$_2$-agonist prn	LA anticholinergic or LA beta$_2$-agonist or SA beta$_2$-agonist and SA anticholinergic	Theophylline
B	LA anticholinergic or LA beta$_2$-agonist	LA anticholinergic and LA beta$_2$-agonist	SA beta$_2$-agonist and/or SA anticholinergic Theophylline
C	ICS + LA beta$_2$-agonist or LA anticholinergic	LA anticholinergic and LA beta$_2$-agonist or LA anticholinergic and PDE-4 Inhibitor or LA beta$_2$-agonist and PDE-4 Inhibitor	SA beta$_2$-agonist and/or SA anticholinergic Theophylline
D	ICS + LA beta$_2$-agonist and/or LA anticholinergic	ICS + LA beta$_2$-agonist and LA anticholinergic or ICS + LA beta$_2$-agonist and PDE-4 inhibitor or LA anticholinergic and LA beta$_2$-agonist or LA anticholinergic and PDE-4 inhibitor	Carbocysteine N-acetylcysteine SA beta$_2$-agonist and/or SA anticholinergic Theophylline

*Medications in each box are mentioned in alphabetical order and therefore not necessarily in order of preference.

**Medications in this column can be used alone or in combination with other options in the First and Alternative Choice columns

Glossary:
SA: short-acting
LA: long-acting
ICS: inhaled corticosteroid
PDE-4: phosphodiesterase-4
prn: when necessary

MANAGEMENT OF EXACERBATIONS

An exacerbation of COPD is defined as **an acute event characterized by a worsening of the patient's respiratory symptoms that is beyond normal day-to-day variations and leads to a change in medication.**

The most common causes appear to be respiratory tract infections (viral or bacterial).

How to Assess the Severity of an Exacerbation

- Arterial blood gas measurements (in hospital): PaO_2 < 8.0 kPa (60 mmHg) with or without $PaCO_2$ > 6.7 kPa, (50 mmHg) when breathing room air indicates respiratory failure.
- Chest radiographs are useful in excluding alternative diagnoses.
- An ECG may aid in the diagnosis of coexisting cardiac problems.

Other laboratory tests:

- *Whole blood count* can identify polycythemia or bleeding.
- The presence of *purulent sputum* during an exacerbation can be sufficient indication for starting empirical antibiotic treatment.
- *Biochemical tests* can help detect electrolyte disturbances, diabetes, and poor nutrition.

Spirometric tests are not recommended during an exacerbation because they can be difficult to perform and measurements are not accurate enough.

Treatment Options

Oxygen: Supplemental oxygen should be titrated to improve the patient's hypoxemia with a target saturation of 88-92%.

Bronchodilators: Short-acting inhaled beta$_2$-agonists with or without short-acting anticholinergics are the preferred bronchodilators for treatment of an exacerbation.

Systemic Corticosteroids: Systemic corticosteroids shorten recovery time, improve lung function (FEV_1) and arterial hypoxemia (PaO_2), and reduce the risks of early relapse, treatment failure, and length of hospital stay. A dose of 40 mg prednisone per day for 5 days is recommended.

Antibiotics: Antibiotics should be given to patients:

- With the following three cardinal symptoms: increased dyspnea, increased sputum volume, increased sputum purulence;
- With increased sputum purulence and one other cardinal symptom;
- Who require mechanical ventilation

Adjunct Therapies: Depending on the clinical condition of the patient, an appropriate fluid balance with special attention to the administration of diuretics, anticoagulants, treatment of comorbidities, and nutritional aspects should be considered. At all times, health care providers should strongly enforce stringent measures against active cigarette smoking. Patients hospitalized because of exacerbations of COPD are at increased risk of deep vein thrombosis and pulmonary embolism; thromboprophylactic measures should be enhanced.

Patients with characteristics of a severe exacerbation should be hospitalized (**Table 8**). Indications for referral and the management of exacerbations of COPD in the hospital depend on local resources and the facilities of the local hospital.

Table 8. Indications for Hospital Assessment or Admission
• Marked increase in intensity of symptoms
• Severe underlying COPD
• Onset of new physical signs
• Failure of an exacerbation to respond to initial medical management
• Presence of serious comorbidities
• Frequent exacerbations
• Older age
• Insufficient home support

COPD AND COMORBIDITIES

COPD often coexists with other diseases (comorbidities) that may have a significant impact on prognosis. In general, the presence of comorbidities should not alter COPD treatment and comorbidities should be treated as if the patient did not have COPD.

Cardiovascular disease (including ischemic heart disease, heart failure, atrial fibrillation, and hypertension) is a major comorbidity in COPD and probably both the most frequent and most important disease coexisting with COPD. Cardioselective beta-blockers are not contraindicated in COPD.

Osteoporosis, anxiety/depression, and **impaired cognitive function,** major comorbidities in COPD, are often under-diagnosed and are associated with poor health status and prognosis.

Lung cancer is frequently seen in patients with COPD and has been found to be the most frequent cause of death in patients with mild COPD.

Serious **infections**, especially respiratory infections, are frequently seen in patients with COPD.

The presence of **metabolic syndrome** and manifest **diabetes** are more frequent in COPD and the latter is likely to impact on prognosis. Gastroesophageal reflux (GERD) is a systemic comorbidity that may have an impact on the lungs.

Increasing use of computed tomography in the assessment of patients with COPD is identifying the presence of previously unrecognized radiographic **bronchiectasis** that appears to be associated with longer exacerbations and increased mortality.

APPENDIX I: SPIROMETRY FOR DIAGNOSIS OF AIRFLOW LIMITATION IN COPD

Spirometry is required to make a clinical diagnosis of COPD and should be available to all health care professionals who work with COPD patients.

What is Spirometry?

Spirometry is a simple test to measure the amount of air a person can breathe out, and the amount of time taken to do so.

A spirometer is a device used to measure how effectively, and how quickly, the lungs can be emptied.

A **spirogram** is a volume-time curve.

Spirometry measurements used for diagnosis of COPD include (see Figures 1A and 1B):

- FVC (Forced Vital Capacity): maximum volume of air that can be exhaled during a forced maneuver.

- FEV_1 (Forced Expired Volume in one second): volume expired in the first second of maximal expiration after a maximal inspiration. This is a measure of how quickly the lungs can be emptied.

- FEV_1/FVC: FEV_1 expressed as a proportion of the FVC, gives a clinically useful index of airflow limitation.

The ratio FEV_1/FVC is between 0.70 and 0.80 in normal adults; a value less than 0.70 indicates airflow limitation and thus of COPD.

FEV_1 is influenced by the age, sex, height, and ethnicity, and is best considered as a percentage of the predicted normal value. There is a vast literature on normal values; those appropriate for local populations should be used[1,2,3,4].

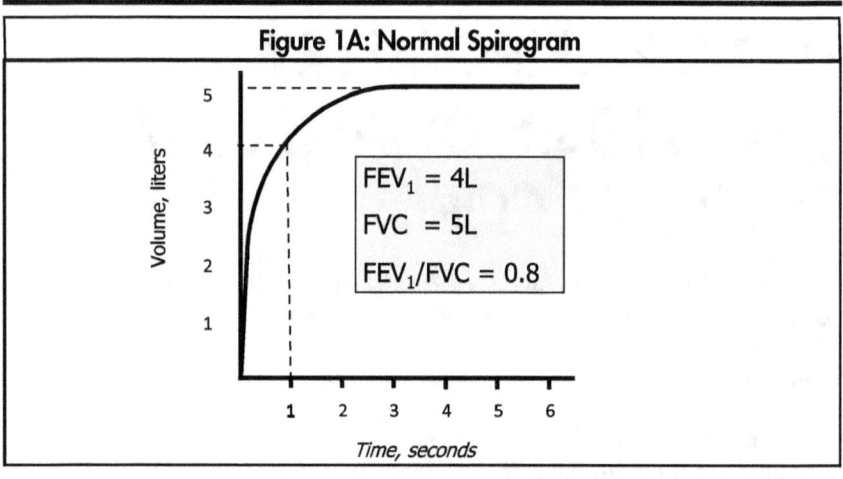

Figure 1A: Normal Spirogram

$FEV_1 = 4L$
$FVC = 5L$
$FEV_1/FVC = 0.8$

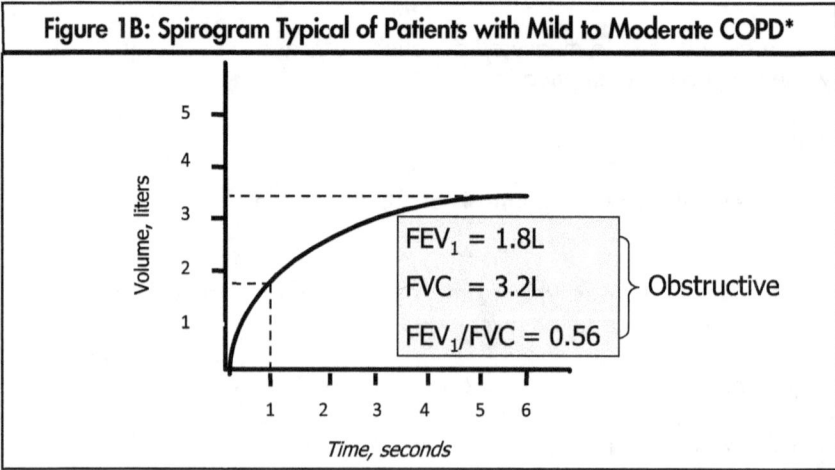

Figure 1B: Spirogram Typical of Patients with Mild to Moderate COPD*

$FEV_1 = 1.8L$
$FVC = 3.2L$
$FEV_1/FVC = 0.56$

Obstructive

Why do Spirometry for COPD?

- Spirometry is needed to make a clinical diagnosis of COPD.

- Together with the presence of symptoms, spirometry helps gauge COPD severity and can be a guide to specific treatment steps.

- A normal value for spirometry effectively excludes the diagnosis of clinically relevant COPD.

- The lower the percentage predicted FEV_1, the worse the subsequent prognosis.

- FEV$_1$ declines over time and usually faster in COPD than in healthy subjects. Spirometry can be used to monitor disease progression, but to be reliable the intervals between measurements must be at least 12 months.

What You Need to Perform Spirometry

Several types of spirometers are available. Relatively large bellows or rolling-seal spirometers are usually only available in pulmonary function laboratories. Calibration should be checked against a known volume (e.g., from a 3-litre syringe) on a regular basis. There are several smaller hand-held devices, often with electronic calibration systems.

A hard copy of the volume-time plot is very useful to checkoptimal performance and interpretation, and to exclude errors.

Most spirometers require electrical power to permit operation of the motor and/or sensors. Some battery-operated versions are available that can dock with a computer to provide hard copy.

It is essential to learn how your machine is calibrated and when and how to clean it.

How to Perform Spirometry

Spirometry is best performed with the patient seated. Patients may be anxious about performing the tests properly, and should be reassured. Careful explanation of the test, accompanied by a demonstration, is very useful. The patient should:

- Breathe in fully.
- Seal their lips around the mouthpiece.
- Force the air out of the chest as hard and fast as they can until their lungs are completely "empty."
- Breathe in again and relax.

Exhalation must continue until no more air can be exhaled, must be at least 6 seconds, and can take up to 15 seconds or more.

Like any test, spirometry results will only be of value if the expirations are performed satisfactorily and consistently. Both FVC and FEV_1 should be the largest value obtained from any of 3 technically satisfactory curves and the FVC and FEV_1 values in these three curves should vary by no more than 5% or 150 ml, whichever is greater. The FEV_1/FVC is calculated using the maximum FEV_1 and FVC from technically acceptable (not necessarily the same) curves.

Those with chest pain or frequent cough may be unable to perform a satisfactory test and this should be noted.

Where to find more detailed information on spirometry:

1. GOLD: A spirometry guide for general practitioners and a teaching slide set is available: http://www.goldcopd.org

2. American Thoracic Society
    http://www.thoracic.org/adobe/statements/spirometry1-30.pdf

3. Australian/New Zealand Thoracic Society
    http://www.nationalasthma.org.au/publications/spiro/index.htm

4. British Thoracic Society
    http://www.brit-thoracic.org.uk/copd/consortium.html

NOTES

NOTES

www.ingramcontent.com/pod-product-compliance
Lightning Source LLC
Chambersburg PA
CBHW070341190526
45169CB00005B/1987